C.S. WALLTER

Guide to become a great Stepfather

I would like to dedicate this book to my own stepdaughter Jessica.
Thank you for putting up with all the trials and tribulations.

To my own stepfather Frank.
Thank you for always being there for me.

Contents

Introduction:

Navigating the intricate terrain of stepfatherhood is a journey filled with challenges, complexities, and heartfelt moments of connection. Understanding the role of a stepfather requires more than just assuming paternal responsibilities; it entails embracing a multifaceted position within the blended family unit. From respecting boundaries to building relationships, establishing trust, and navigating challenges, the role of a stepfather encompasses a myriad of responsibilities that shape the dynamics and wellbeing of the family.

In this exploration of stepfatherhood,, we gain a deeper understanding of the joys and struggles that define the role of a stepfather, as well as the profound impact it has on both the individual and the family as a whole.

Throughout this journey, you will embody the essence of stepfatherhood with unwavering dedication, compassion, and resilience. Their experiences serve as a testament to the profound bonds that can be forged within blended families, and the transformative power of love, patience, and understanding in navigating the complexities of stepfatherhood.

As we embark on this exploration of the role of a stepfather, we invite you to join us on a journey of discovery, reflection, and insight into the challenges, triumphs, and profound moments of connection that define the essence of stepfatherhood. Through our shared experiences, we hope to gain a deeper appreciation for the role of a stepfather and the invaluable contributions they make to the lives of their stepchildren and the blended family unit as a whole.

Section 1: Understanding the Role of a Stepfather: Chapter 1: Embracing your Role

Becoming a stepfather is a significant life transition that brings both challenges and rewards. Unlike biological fatherhood, stepfatherhood comes with its own unique set of dynamics and responsibilities. Understanding the role of a stepfather and embracing it wholeheartedly is essential for building strong and meaningful relationships within the blended family unit.

The role of a stepfather encompasses more than just providing financial support or acting as a disciplinarian. It involves assuming a nurturing and supportive role in the lives of your stepchildren, contributing to their emotional well-being, and serving as a positive role model and mentor. Embracing the role of a stepfather means recognizing the importance of your presence in your stepchildren's lives and actively participating in their upbringing and development.

One of the key aspects of embracing the role of a stepfather is understanding the unique dynamics of blended families. Blended families often come with their own set of challenges, such as adjusting to new family dynamics, navigating relationships with biological parents, and managing expectations. As a stepfather, it is essential to approach these challenges with patience, empathy, and understanding. Building trust and rapport with your stepchildren takes time and effort, but it is crucial for fostering a strong and harmonious family dynamic.

Embracing the role of a stepfather also means recognizing and respecting the boundaries and preferences of your stepchildren. Every child is unique, with their own personality, interests, and needs. It is essential to acknowledge and respect these differences and to tailor your approach to parenting accordingly. Taking the time to get to know your stepchildren on an individual level, listening to their thoughts and feelings, and supporting their interests and aspirations can help strengthen your bond and build trust and respect within the family.

Another important aspect of embracing the role of a stepfather is fostering open communication within the blended family unit. Effective communication is key to resolving conflicts, addressing concerns, and building strong relationships. Creating a safe and supportive environment where your stepchildren feel comfortable expressing themselves and sharing their thoughts and feelings is essential for fostering trust and mutual respect.

Embracing the role of a stepfather also involves acknowledging and celebrating the milestones and achievements of your stepchildren. Whether it's a graduation, a sports victory, or a personal accomplishment, taking the time to acknowledge and celebrate these moments helps reinforce your support and encouragement and strengthens your bond with your stepchildren.

Chapter 2: Open Communication

Open communication is a cornerstone of successful stepfatherhood. As a stepfather, fostering an environment where communication flows freely is essential for building trust, strengthening relationships, and navigating the complexities of blended family dynamics. Understanding the role of open communication in stepfatherhood and embracing it wholeheartedly can lead to healthier and more fulfilling family relationships.

One of the key aspects of open communication as a stepfather is creating a safe and supportive space where your stepchildren feel comfortable expressing themselves. Blended families often come with their own set of challenges, including adjusting to new family dynamics and navigating relationships with biological parents. By encouraging open communication, you provide your stepchildren with an outlet to voice their thoughts, feelings, and concerns, helping them feel heard and validated.

Building trust is another important aspect of open communication in stepfatherhood. Trust is the foundation of any healthy relationship, and fostering open communication helps build trust between you and your stepchildren. By being honest, transparent, and reliable in your interactions with your stepchildren, you demonstrate your trustworthiness and reliability, laying the groundwork for stronger and more meaningful relationships.

Open communication also plays a vital role in resolving conflicts and addressing concerns within the blended family unit. Conflicts are a natural part of family life, and learning to navigate them constructively is essential for maintaining harmony and unity within the family. By fostering open communication, you create an environment where conflicts can be addressed openly and honestly, allowing for the resolution of issues in a respectful and constructive manner.

As a stepfather, it is important to lead by example when it comes to open communication. Modeling effective communication skills, such as active listening, empathy, and understanding, sets a positive example for your stepchildren and encourages them to communicate openly and honestly with you and other family members. By demonstrating a willingness to listen and understand your stepchildren's perspectives, you show them that their thoughts and feelings are valued and respected.

Embracing open communication as a stepfather also involves being proactive in initiating conversations and checking in with your stepchildren regularly. Taking the time to engage in meaningful conversations with your stepchildren, whether it's over dinner or during family activities, helps strengthen your bond and build trust. By showing a genuine interest in your stepchildren's lives and experiences, you create opportunities for deeper connection and understanding.

Chapter 3: Respect Boundaries

Respecting boundaries is a fundamental aspect of stepfatherhood, crucial for building trust, fostering healthy relationships, and creating a supportive family environment. As a stepfather, understanding the importance of respecting boundaries and embracing this role with empathy and sensitivity is essential for navigating the complexities of blended family dynamics.

One of the primary aspects of respecting boundaries as a stepfather is acknowledging and understanding the individual boundaries and preferences of your stepchildren. Every child is unique, with their own set of boundaries, likes, dislikes, and personal space. Recognizing and respecting these boundaries demonstrates your respect for your stepchildren's autonomy and helps foster trust and mutual respect within the family.

Respecting boundaries also involves acknowledging the role of the biological parents in the lives of your stepchildren. While you may play a significant role in your stepchildren's upbringing, it is essential to recognize and respect the authority and preferences of the biological parents. Co-parenting with sensitivity and respect means understanding and adhering to the boundaries set by the biological parents, whether it's regarding discipline, decision-making, or parenting styles.

Creating an open dialogue with your stepchildren about boundaries is another important aspect of stepfatherhood. Encouraging your stepchildren to express their boundaries, preferences, and concerns openly helps create a safe and supportive environment where their voices are heard and respected. By actively listening to your stepchildren's needs and concerns, you demonstrate your willingness to understand and accommodate their boundaries, fostering trust and mutual respect in your relationship.

Respecting boundaries also extends to your own actions and behaviors as a stepfather. Setting appropriate boundaries for yourself, such as respecting your stepchildren's privacy, avoiding intrusive questions, and refraining from imposing your own expectations or beliefs, is essential for building trust and maintaining healthy relationships within the blended family unit. By modeling respectful behavior and boundaries, you provide your stepchildren with a positive example to follow and create a supportive family environment where everyone's boundaries are respected.

Navigating boundaries within the blended family unit may also require flexibility and adaptability. As family dynamics evolve and relationships develop over time, it is essential to remain open to adjusting boundaries and accommodating changing needs and preferences. Being receptive to feedback from your stepchildren and other family members and willing to make adjustments as necessary demonstrates your commitment to creating a harmonious and supportive family environment.

Section 2: Building Relationships:
Chapter 4: Take Your Time

Becoming a stepfather is a journey that requires patience, understanding, and a willingness to adapt to new family dynamics. Understanding the role of a stepfather means recognizing that building relationships and integrating into a blended family takes time. Embracing patience and understanding is essential for navigating the complexities of stepfatherhood and creating a supportive and harmonious family environment.

One of the most important aspects of understanding the role of a stepfather is recognizing that relationships cannot be rushed. Building trust and rapport with stepchildren, establishing a bond with your partner, and navigating co-parenting dynamics all take time and patience. Rushing these processes can lead to misunderstandings, resentment, and strained relationships. Embracing patience means allowing relationships to develop organically and being willing to invest the time and effort necessary to build strong and meaningful connections with your stepchildren and other family members.

Understanding the role of a stepfather also means recognizing and accepting that blending families comes with its own set of challenges and adjustments. As a stepfather, you may encounter resistance, confusion, or uncertainty from your stepchildren as they adjust to their new family dynamic. Embracing patience and understanding means approaching these challenges with empathy and compassion, acknowledging the emotions and concerns of your stepchildren, and providing reassurance and support as they navigate the transition.

Patience and understanding are also essential when it comes to navigating co-parenting dynamics with the biological parents. Co-parenting requires effective communication, compromise, and flexibility, all of which take time to develop. Embracing patience means being willing to listen to the perspectives and preferences of the biological parents, respecting their authority and decisions regarding their children, and working together collaboratively to ensure the well-being of the entire family unit.

Taking your time as a stepfather also means being patient with yourself. Adjusting to your new role within the blended family may take time, and it's okay to make mistakes along the way. Embracing patience means allowing yourself grace and understanding as you navigate the challenges and uncertainties of stepfatherhood, seeking support and guidance when needed, and being willing to learn and grow from your experiences.

Chapter 5: Shared Activities

Shared activities play a pivotal role in the journey of stepfatherhood, providing opportunities for bonding, creating lasting memories, and fostering strong relationships within the blended family. Understanding the significance of shared activities and embracing them as a stepfather is essential for building trust, strengthening connections, and nurturing a sense of belonging among family members.

One of the most effective ways for stepfathers to bond with their stepchildren is through shared activities that cater to mutual interests and hobbies. Whether it's playing sports together, engaging in outdoor adventures, or pursuing creative endeavors, finding common ground and participating in activities that resonate with both the stepfather and stepchildren can create opportunities for meaningful interaction and bonding. Embracing shared activities allows stepfathers to connect with their stepchildren on a personal level, fostering a sense of camaraderie and building trust and rapport over time.

Shared activities also provide a platform for stepfathers to demonstrate their support and encouragement for their stepchildren's interests and passions. By actively participating in activities that are important to their stepchildren, stepfathers show that they value and respect their individuality and are invested in their happiness and well-being. Whether it's attending a dance recital, cheering on a sports game, or helping with a school project, being present and engaged in their stepchildren's lives through shared activities strengthens the bond between stepfather and stepchild and fosters a sense of mutual appreciation and respect.

In addition to bonding with stepchildren, shared activities also offer opportunities for stepfathers to nurture their relationship with their partner. Engaging in shared activities as a family unit allows stepfathers and their partners to create cherished memories together and strengthen their connection as a couple. Whether it's going on family outings, planning vacations, or simply spending quality time together at home, shared activities reinforce the foundation of love and commitment within the blended family and contribute to a sense of unity and cohesiveness.

Embracing shared activities as a stepfather also means being flexible and open-minded when it comes to exploring new experiences and interests with your stepchildren. While it's important to engage in activities that resonate with both the stepfather and stepchildren, it's also valuable to step out of your comfort zone and try new things together. Whether it's learning a new hobby, exploring a new destination, or embarking on a family adventure, stepping outside of familiar routines and embracing new experiences fosters growth, learning, and mutual appreciation within the blended family.

Chapter 6: Support the Biological Parent

Supporting the biological parent is a crucial aspect of stepfatherhood, as it fosters unity, strengthens relationships, and promotes the well-being of the entire family unit. Understanding the importance of supporting the biological parent and embracing this role with empathy and compassion is essential for creating a supportive and harmonious blended family environment.

One of the primary responsibilities of a stepfather is to support and respect the authority of the biological parent. While stepfathers play an integral role in the lives of their stepchildren, it is essential to recognize that the biological parent holds a unique and irreplaceable position in their children's lives. Embracing the role of supporting the biological parent means acknowledging their authority and decision-making power regarding their children and respecting their role as the primary caregiver.

Supporting the biological parent also involves fostering open communication and collaboration in co-parenting efforts. Effective co-parenting requires clear communication, mutual respect, and a willingness to work together in the best interests of the children. As a stepfather, it is essential to approach co-parenting with empathy and understanding, listening to the perspectives and concerns of the biological parent, and actively participating in discussions and decision-making processes regarding the upbringing of the children.

Embracing the role of supporting the biological parent also means providing emotional and practical support in times of need. Parenting can be challenging, and offering a listening ear, a shoulder to lean on, or a helping hand can make a significant difference to the biological parent. Whether it's offering encouragement during difficult times, helping with household chores or childcare responsibilities, or simply being a supportive presence, stepfathers can play a vital role in alleviating the stresses and burdens faced by the biological parent.

Supporting the biological parent also involves fostering a positive relationship between the biological parent and their children. Encouraging and facilitating regular communication, fostering a sense of trust and mutual respect, and promoting quality time spent together as a family unit strengthens the bond between the biological parent and their children and reinforces their authority and role within the family.

In addition to supporting the biological parent, it is also essential for stepfathers to prioritize their own relationship with their partner. Nurturing a strong and healthy relationship with their partner lays the foundation for a supportive and harmonious blended family environment. By communicating openly, expressing appreciation and affection, and working together as a team, stepfathers and their partners create a stable and loving home environment where all family members feel valued, respected, and supported.

Section 3 Establishing Trust: Chapter 7: Be Reliable

Reliability is a cornerstone of stepfatherhood, playing a crucial role in building trust, fostering stability, and nurturing strong relationships within the blended family unit. Understanding the importance of being reliable and embracing this role with dedication and consistency is essential for creating a supportive and harmonious family environment.

As a stepfather, being reliable means demonstrating consistency and dependability in your words and actions. Consistency provides a sense of stability and predictability for your stepchildren, helping them feel secure and supported within the blended family unit. Whether it's fulfilling promises, following through on commitments, or being present for important milestones and events, being reliable establishes trust and reinforces your role as a supportive and caring figure in your stepchildren's lives.

Embracing the role of being reliable also involves prioritizing the well-being and needs of your stepchildren. Being available and responsive to their emotional and practical needs fosters a sense of trust and security within the family. Whether it's offering a listening ear, providing guidance and support, or being a source of encouragement during challenging times, being reliable means being there for your stepchildren consistently, regardless of the circumstances.

Reliability is especially crucial when it comes to co-parenting with the biological parent. Collaborative co-parenting requires effective communication, mutual respect, and a commitment to working together in the best interests of the children. Being reliable in co-parenting efforts means honoring agreements, respecting boundaries, and prioritizing the needs of the children above all else. By demonstrating reliability in co-parenting, stepfathers contribute to a supportive and cohesive co-parenting relationship that benefits the entire family unit.

In addition to being reliable in day-to-day interactions, stepfathers can also demonstrate their reliability through their commitment to their role within the blended family. Embracing the responsibilities of stepfatherhood with dedication and consistency reinforces your commitment to the well-being and happiness of your stepchildren. Whether it's taking on parenting responsibilities, participating in family activities, or contributing to household chores and responsibilities, being reliable means showing up for your family consistently and wholeheartedly.

Being reliable also involves being honest and transparent in your communication with your stepchildren. Building trust requires open and honest communication, and being reliable means being truthful and forthcoming in your interactions with your stepchildren. By communicating openly and authentically, stepfathers foster trust and mutual respect within the blended family unit, creating a supportive and nurturing environment where everyone feels valued and respected.

Chapter 8: Respect the Child's Privacy

Respecting the privacy of stepchildren is a fundamental aspect of stepfatherhood, crucial for building trust, fostering mutual respect, and nurturing healthy relationships within the blended family unit. Understanding the importance of respecting the child's privacy and embracing this role with empathy and sensitivity is essential for creating a supportive and harmonious family environment.

One of the primary responsibilities of a stepfather is to create a safe and secure environment where stepchildren feel respected and valued. Respecting the child's privacy means recognizing their right to autonomy and personal space, and refraining from intruding into areas that they consider private or off-limits. Whether it's respecting their physical boundaries, such as knocking before entering their room, or respecting their emotional boundaries, such as refraining from prying into personal matters, respecting the child's privacy demonstrates your commitment to their well-being and reinforces your role as a supportive and respectful figure in their lives.

Respecting the child's privacy also involves being mindful of their need for independence and autonomy. As stepchildren navigate the challenges of adolescence and young adulthood, it is essential to give them space to explore their identities, make their own choices, and develop a sense of autonomy. Embracing the role of respecting the child's privacy means supporting their independence, respecting their decisions, and providing guidance and support when needed, without imposing your own expectations or agendas onto them.

In addition to respecting physical and emotional boundaries, stepfathers can also demonstrate their respect for the child's privacy through their actions and behaviors. Being mindful of the child's need for confidentiality and discretion, refraining from sharing personal information or sensitive topics without their consent, and respecting their right to privacy in digital spaces, such as social media and electronic devices, are all important ways to show respect for the child's privacy and foster trust and mutual respect within the blended family unit.

Respecting the child's privacy also involves fostering open communication and trust within the family. Creating an environment where stepchildren feel comfortable expressing themselves, sharing their thoughts and feelings, and seeking support and guidance when needed, reinforces their sense of autonomy and independence. By listening actively, validating their experiences, and respecting their boundaries, stepfathers can create a supportive and nurturing family environment where stepchildren feel valued and respected.

Chapter 9: Be Patient

Patience is not merely a virtue; it's a cornerstone of successful stepfatherhood. Navigating the intricate paths of blended families requires a steadfast commitment to patience—an attribute that fosters understanding, resilience, and ultimately, enduring bonds. In comprehending the pivotal role patience plays, stepfathers can cultivate a nurturing and supportive environment where love, trust, and respect thrive.

At the heart of stepfatherhood lies the necessity to recognize that relationships need time to blossom. Unlike biological bonds, which often grow from infancy, stepfather-stepchild relationships evolve from unfamiliar territory. Patience becomes the guiding force as stepfathers embark on the journey of building connections, allowing trust to sprout gradually through shared experiences and heartfelt conversations. Each moment of patience invested lays the foundation for deeper, more meaningful relationships.

Embracing patience also entails navigating the ebb and flow of emotions within the blended family unit. Stepfathers may encounter resistance, hesitation, or even resentment from stepchildren as they adjust to the new family dynamic. In these moments, patience serves as a beacon of understanding, providing space for stepchildren to process their feelings and acclimate to their new reality. By demonstrating patience and empathy, stepfathers pave the way for healing and growth, fostering an environment where stepchildren feel heard, supported, and accepted.

Patience extends beyond individual relationships to encompass the broader dynamics of co-parenting and family integration. Collaborative efforts between stepfathers and biological parents require time, communication, and compromise to flourish. Embracing patience means navigating co-parenting challenges with grace and understanding, acknowledging the complexities of blended family life, and working together to prioritize the well-being of the children above all else. Through patience and cooperation, stepfathers can forge strong partnerships with biological parents, fostering unity and harmony within the family unit.

In addition to fostering external relationships, patience plays a pivotal role in nurturing self-growth and resilience within stepfathers themselves. Adjusting to the demands of stepfatherhood requires a willingness to learn, adapt, and grow over time. Patience allows stepfathers to navigate setbacks and challenges with resilience, recognizing that progress is often incremental and success is measured not by speed, but by steadfast dedication and perseverance.

Section 4 Navigating Challenges: Chapter 10: Handle Discipline with Care

Discipline is a delicate aspect of stepfatherhood, requiring a balance of authority and empathy to foster growth and harmony within the blended family unit. Understanding the nuances of discipline and embracing this role with care and sensitivity is essential for nurturing positive relationships and creating a supportive environment where stepchildren feel respected and understood.

At the core of effective discipline lies the importance of consistency and fairness. Stepfathers must establish clear boundaries and expectations, ensuring that rules are communicated openly and enforced consistently. By setting clear guidelines and adhering to them fairly, stepfathers create a sense of structure and security within the family, helping stepchildren understand their roles and responsibilities while fostering respect for authority.

However, discipline in the context of stepfatherhood requires a nuanced approach that takes into account the unique dynamics of blended families. Stepfathers must navigate the complexities of stepchildren's relationships with their biological parents, recognizing that discipline is a shared responsibility that requires collaboration and mutual respect. By consulting with the biological parent and aligning on disciplinary strategies, stepfathers can ensure that disciplinary measures are consistent and cohesive, promoting unity and harmony within the family unit.

Embracing the role of handling discipline with care also entails understanding the underlying motivations behind misbehavior. Stepfathers must approach discipline with empathy and understanding, recognizing that misbehavior may stem from a variety of factors, including adjustment issues, emotional distress, or feelings of insecurity. By addressing underlying issues with compassion and support, rather than punitive measures, stepfathers can help stepchildren feel heard and understood, fostering trust and strengthening their bond over time.

Moreover, discipline in stepfatherhood necessitates a focus on positive reinforcement and encouragement. While consequences for misbehavior are important, stepfathers should also prioritize opportunities to praise and reward positive behavior. By acknowledging and celebrating stepchildren's achievements and efforts, stepfathers reinforce desired behaviors and cultivate a supportive environment where stepchildren feel valued and appreciated.

Handling discipline with care also involves recognizing the importance of open communication and dialogue. Stepfathers should create opportunities for stepchildren to express their thoughts and feelings openly, providing a safe space for them to voice concerns or seek guidance. By fostering open lines of communication, stepfathers demonstrate their commitment to understanding stepchildren's perspectives and concerns, building trust and mutual respect within the family.

Chapter 11: Address Jealousy and Resentment

Jealousy and resentment can be formidable obstacles in the journey of stepfatherhood, posing challenges to building trust, fostering positive relationships, and creating a harmonious family environment. Understanding the complexities of these emotions and embracing strategies to address them with empathy and sensitivity is essential for nurturing strong bonds and promoting unity within the blended family unit.

One of the most common sources of jealousy and resentment in stepfather-stepchild relationships stems from feelings of displacement and insecurity. Stepchildren may experience jealousy towards their stepfather, fearing that their bond with their biological parent will be compromised or overshadowed. Similarly, stepfathers may grapple with feelings of resentment towards their stepchildren, particularly if they perceive them as obstacles to their relationship with their partner or if they feel excluded or undervalued within the family.

Addressing jealousy and resentment begins with open and honest communication. Stepfathers and stepchildren should have opportunities to express their thoughts and feelings openly, creating a safe space for dialogue and understanding. By acknowledging and validating each other's perspectives, stepfathers and stepchildren can work towards resolving underlying issues and building trust and mutual respect within the family.

Empathy plays a crucial role in addressing jealousy and resentment in stepfather-stepchild relationships. Stepfathers must strive to understand the root causes of their stepchildren's feelings, recognizing that jealousy and resentment often stem from fears of abandonment, loss, or rejection. By demonstrating empathy and compassion, stepfathers can reassure their stepchildren of their love and commitment, helping to alleviate feelings of insecurity and fostering a sense of belonging within the family.

Similarly, stepfathers may experience feelings of resentment towards their stepchildren, particularly if they perceive them as disruptive or challenging to their relationship with their partner. In these instances, it is essential for stepfathers to acknowledge and process their emotions constructively, seeking support from their partner or a trusted confidant if needed. By addressing their feelings of resentment with honesty and vulnerability, stepfathers can work towards fostering healthier and more positive relationships with their stepchildren.

Building trust and rapport is paramount in addressing jealousy and resentment within the blended family unit. Stepfathers must demonstrate their commitment to their stepchildren's well-being and happiness through their actions and behaviors. By investing time and effort in building meaningful connections, participating in shared activities, and providing emotional support, stepfathers can earn their stepchildren's trust and respect, fostering stronger and more resilient relationships over time.

Chapter 12: Seek Professional Guidance if Needed

Navigating the multifaceted role of a stepfather often presents challenges that may require additional support and guidance. Seeking professional guidance is a proactive approach that can provide stepfathers with valuable insights, tools, and strategies to address complex family dynamics, foster positive relationships, and promote the well-being of everyone involved. Understanding the importance of seeking professional guidance and embracing this role with openness and receptivity is essential for creating a supportive and nurturing family environment within the blended family unit.

One of the primary benefits of seeking professional guidance is gaining access to expert knowledge and experience in navigating blended family dynamics. Family therapists, counselors, and other mental health professionals specialize in addressing the unique challenges faced by blended families, offering tailored strategies and interventions to help stepfathers and their families overcome obstacles and build strong, resilient relationships. By leveraging the expertise of these professionals, stepfathers can gain valuable insights into effective communication techniques, conflict resolution strategies, and co-parenting approaches that promote harmony and unity within the family unit.

Seeking professional guidance also provides a safe and confidential space for stepfathers to explore and address personal and relational challenges. Family therapy sessions offer stepfathers and their families an opportunity to express their thoughts and feelings openly, without fear of judgment or criticism. Through guided discussions and therapeutic exercises, stepfathers can gain a deeper understanding of their emotions, beliefs, and behaviors, identify areas for growth and improvement, and develop practical skills and strategies to navigate the complexities of stepfatherhood with confidence and resilience.

Moreover, professional guidance can play a crucial role in facilitating healthy communication and conflict resolution within the blended family unit. Family therapists and counselors specialize in helping stepfathers and their families navigate difficult conversations, manage conflicts constructively, and develop effective problem-solving skills. By learning to communicate openly and respectfully, stepfathers can foster trust, mutual respect, and understanding within the family, laying the groundwork for stronger and more resilient relationships.

In addition to addressing immediate challenges, seeking professional guidance can also provide stepfathers with long-term support and resources to navigate the evolving dynamics of blended family life. Family therapists and counselors can offer ongoing support and guidance as stepfathers and their families adjust to new roles, transitions, and life events, helping them navigate challenges and capitalize on opportunities for growth and connection. By establishing a collaborative relationship with a trusted mental health professional, stepfathers can access a wealth of resources, support networks, and therapeutic interventions to support their journey of stepfatherhood and promote the well-being of their families.

Section 5: Celebrating Achievements: Chapter 13: Acknowledge Milestones

In the intricate tapestry of stepfatherhood, acknowledging and celebrating milestones holds profound significance. These moments serve as poignant reminders of growth, resilience, and the bonds forged within the blended family unit. Understanding the importance of acknowledging milestones and embracing this role with sincerity and enthusiasm is essential for fostering a sense of belonging, strengthening relationships, and creating cherished memories that endure a lifetime.

Milestones come in various forms, ranging from birthdays and graduations to personal achievements and significant life events. Each milestone represents a unique opportunity for stepfathers to demonstrate their love, support, and pride in their stepchildren's accomplishments. By acknowledging these milestones with heartfelt sincerity and enthusiasm, stepfathers validate the efforts and achievements of their stepchildren, instilling a sense of confidence, self-worth, and belonging within the family.

One of the most meaningful ways stepfathers can acknowledge milestones is through personalized gestures and expressions of appreciation. Whether it's writing a heartfelt letter, creating a handmade gift, or planning a special outing or celebration, stepfathers can demonstrate their genuine interest and investment in their stepchildren's lives, fostering a sense of connection and intimacy that strengthens their bond over time. By acknowledging milestones with thoughtfulness and creativity, stepfathers create lasting memories and traditions that hold deep emotional significance for their stepchildren and the entire family.

Acknowledging milestones also involves being present and engaged in the moment, actively participating in celebrations and commemorations with enthusiasm and genuine interest. By attending school events, sporting competitions, and extracurricular activities, stepfathers demonstrate their unwavering support and encouragement for their stepchildren's passions and pursuits, fostering a sense of pride and accomplishment within the family. By celebrating milestones together, stepfathers and their families create cherished memories and shared experiences that strengthen their bond and deepen their connection with one another.

Moreover, acknowledging milestones provides stepfathers with an opportunity to reflect on the progress and growth achieved within the blended family unit. Celebrating milestones allows stepfathers to acknowledge the resilience and strength demonstrated by their stepchildren and the entire family as they navigate the challenges and triumphs of blended family life. By acknowledging milestones with gratitude and humility, stepfathers honor the collective journey of growth and transformation, fostering a sense of unity, resilience, and shared purpose within the family.

Chapter 14: Create Family Traditions

Family traditions serve as the glue that binds together the intricate fabric of blended families, fostering unity, connection, and a sense of belonging. Understanding the significance of creating and upholding family traditions, and embracing this role with creativity and dedication, is essential for nurturing strong bonds and cultivating cherished memories within the blended family unit.

Family traditions come in various forms, ranging from simple rituals and routines to elaborate celebrations and rituals. Whether it's a weekly game night, a monthly movie marathon, or an annual holiday gathering, these traditions provide opportunities for stepfathers and their families to come together, connect, and create lasting memories. By establishing and upholding family traditions, stepfathers can foster a sense of stability and continuity within the blended family unit, providing a source of comfort and familiarity amidst the complexities of blended family life.

One of the most meaningful aspects of creating family traditions is the opportunity to tailor them to the unique interests and preferences of the blended family members. Stepfathers can collaborate with their partners and stepchildren to brainstorm ideas for new traditions or adapt existing ones to reflect the diverse backgrounds and experiences of everyone involved. By involving stepchildren in the creation and implementation of family traditions, stepfathers empower them to take ownership of their family's culture and heritage, fostering a sense of pride and belonging within the family.

Moreover, creating family traditions provides stepfathers with an opportunity to bond with their stepchildren and strengthen their relationships over time. Whether it's cooking a favorite meal together, embarking on a family adventure, or participating in a shared hobby or activity, engaging in family traditions allows stepfathers to connect with their stepchildren on a deeper level, fostering trust, mutual respect, and understanding. By prioritizing quality time spent together and creating opportunities for meaningful interaction and bonding, stepfathers can build strong and enduring relationships with their stepchildren that withstand the test of time.

In addition to strengthening relationships within the blended family unit, family traditions also provide opportunities for personal growth and reflection. By participating in traditions that honor family values, celebrate milestones, or commemorate special occasions, stepfathers and their families can cultivate a sense of gratitude, appreciation, and mindfulness. By creating moments of shared joy, laughter, and connection, family traditions help foster a positive and nurturing family environment where everyone feels valued, respected, and loved.

Conclusion

In the intricate journey of stepfatherhood, understanding the multifaceted role plays a pivotal role in nurturing thriving blended families. Firstly, comprehending the role entails recognizing the complexities and responsibilities that come with stepping into a paternal figure position. This understanding sets the foundation for respectful and empathetic interactions.

Respecting boundaries is equally vital; acknowledging the autonomy and emotional space of both stepchildren and biological parents fosters trust and cultivates healthy relationships. By maintaining clear communication and demonstrating empathy, stepfathers establish a supportive environment where everyone feels valued and respected.

Building relationships is a continuous process that requires patience, sincerity, and genuine effort. Stepfathers can strengthen bonds by engaging in shared activities, actively listening to their stepchildren's concerns, and being present in their lives. Through consistent and compassionate interactions, stepfathers lay the groundwork for meaningful connections that endure the test of time.

Establishing trust is fundamental in navigating the complexities of blended family dynamics. By demonstrating reliability, consistency, and honesty, stepfathers create a sense of security and stability within the family unit. Trust serves as the cornerstone for effective communication, conflict resolution, and mutual respect, fostering a supportive environment where relationships thrive.

Navigating challenges is an inevitable aspect of stepfatherhood; however, with resilience and perseverance, obstacles can be overcome. By approaching difficulties with patience, understanding, and a willingness to seek support when needed, stepfathers can navigate through turbulent times and emerge stronger as a family unit.

Celebrating achievements is a powerful way to reinforce positive behaviors and strengthen family bonds. By acknowledging and commemorating milestones, both big and small, stepfathers demonstrate their pride and support for their stepchildren's accomplishments. Celebrations serve as opportunities for joy, reflection, and unity, creating cherished memories that bind the family together.

In conclusion, understanding the role of a stepfather encompasses a range of responsibilities, from respecting boundaries to celebrating achievements. By embracing these aspects with empathy, patience, and dedication, stepfathers can nurture thriving blended families built on a foundation of love, trust, and mutual respect. Through continuous effort and unwavering commitment, stepfathers play a vital role in creating a supportive and harmonious family environment where everyone feels valued, understood, and appreciated.